Low Cholesterol Recipes Cookbook

Tasty Low Cholesterol Recipes to Eat Your Way to Health

Table of Contents

Introduction

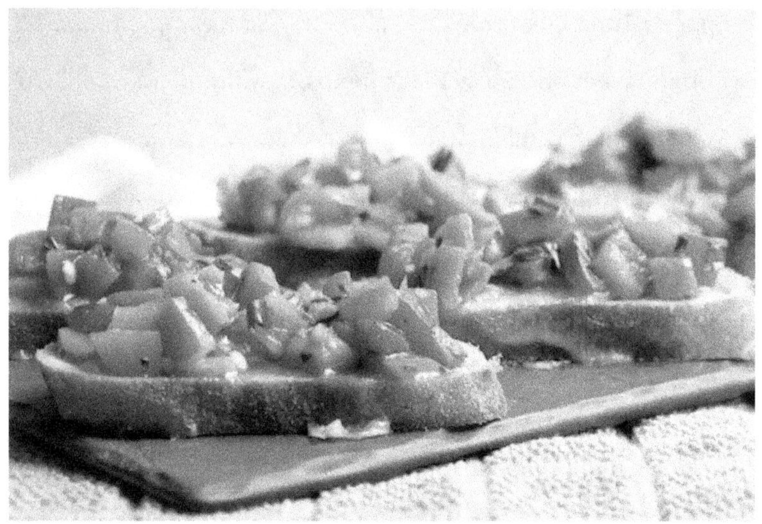

Eating heart-healthy foods never appeals to many because it can lead to meals that are bland and unappetizing. Here we have 30 low cholesterol recipes that will change that myth and deliver some tasty appetizer main meals and a couple of desserts. Anyone who struggles to keep to a healthy diet needs to check out these flavorful dishes which come from many different countries.

Each one is chosen because of the minimal effects on raising cholesterol, and when used as part of your ongoing healthy eating plan, they can help reduce these levels and make you feel healthier overall. In these delicious recipes, you won't find unhealthy fats, trans fats, or anything else which is unhealthy. Only the freshest ingredients are used along with some of the best spices to transform any meal throughout the day into something unique.

It doesn't matter what time of day, or even if you have a gathering of friends or family, you can still enjoy a large meal without worrying. Our top low cholesterol recipes make things easier, and more enjoyable than you could imagine.

Appetizers

Winter Spiced Honey Granola Bars

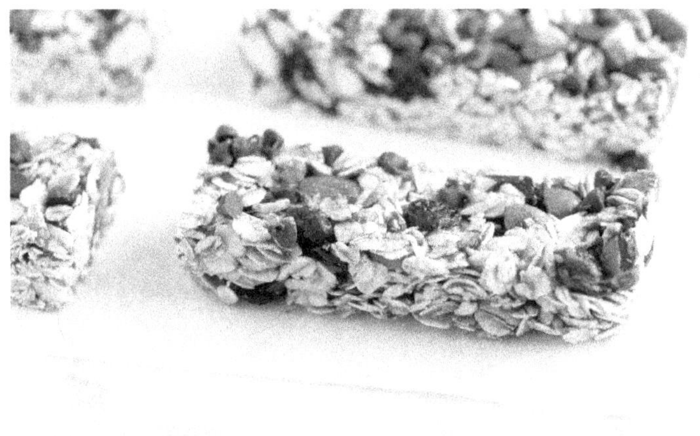

Here is a real energy-boosting bar that packs a hint of spice, a sweet honey flavor, and to spice it up, even more, is the addition of the cocoa powder. You can also make double the batch and make half with the cocoa and half without to keep the kid's in the family happy.

Serving Size: 12

Preparation: 20 minutes

Cooking Time: 20 minutes

Ingredients

- 1 cup of quick-cooking oats
- 1 x large egg
- 1/2 cup of raisins
- 1/2 cup of applesauce
- 1/3 cup of honey
- 1/4 cup of wheat germ
- 1/4 cup of whole-wheat flour
- 1/4 cup of all-purpose flour
- 1 1/2 tbsps. of brown sugar
- 2 tbsps. of unsweetened cocoa powder – can be made with or without
- 1 tsp. of ground cinnamon
- 1 tsp. of ground ginger
- 1/2 tsp. of ground all-spice
- 1/2 tsp. of sea salt
- 1 1/2 tsp. of vanilla extract

Instructions

1. Pre-heat an oven to 350 degrees Fahrenheit

2. Line an 8-inch x 8-inch baking pan with oven-proof parchment paper

3. In a large mixing bowl, add the oats, raisins, both flours, wheat germ, cocoa powder (if using), brown sugar, allspice, cinnamon, ginger, and the salt. Make a hole in the center

4. Whisk in another bowl the applesauce, egg, honey, and the vanilla until well combined

5. Pour this mixture into the hole of the dry **Ingredients**

6. Mix using two spoons until thoroughly mixed

7. Once mixed, pour the batter into lined baking pan and press flat

8. Place into the preheated oven and bake for 20-minutes or until firm

9. Once cooked, remove from pan and cool for 10-minutes

10. Slice into 12 equal pieces

Roasted Red Pepper Bruschetta

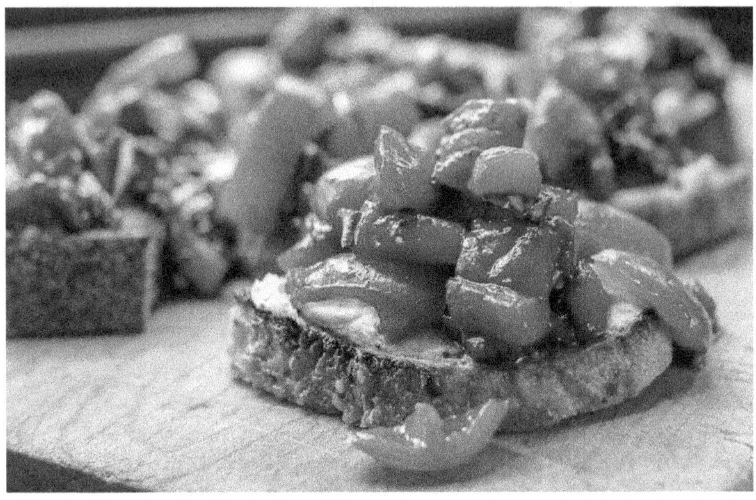

When you have a family dinner or friends around, there is nothing as quick and easy, never mind tasty as the delicious bite-sized Bruschetta slices topped with roasted red peppers with a hint of garlic and a lashing of tasty extra virgin olive oil.

Serving Size: 12

Preparation: 5 minutes

Cooking Time: 5 minutes

Ingredients

- 16 oz. of Italian Bruschetta
- 2 tbsps. of virgin olive oil
- 1 x 16 oz. jar of roasted red peppers. Sweet variety
- 1 large onion, coarsely chopped
- 1 large tomato, remove seeds and chop roughly
- 3 x garlic cloves, finely chopped
- 1 cup of fresh basil coarsely chopped
- 3 tsp. of balsamic vinegar

Instructions

1. Preheat the oven broiler.

2. Slice the bread into slices around 1-inch thick.

3. Brush one side with olive oil.

4. Broil with the oil-side face-up. Cook until lightly golden.

5. Remove from the broiler and set aside.

6. Add to a medium mixing bowl the roasted peppers, tomato, garlic, onion, and the chopped basil.

7. Mix to combine and then top each bread slice with mixture.

8. Drizzle with a little of the balsamic vinegar and serve immediately.

Grill Fired Oyster Shooters

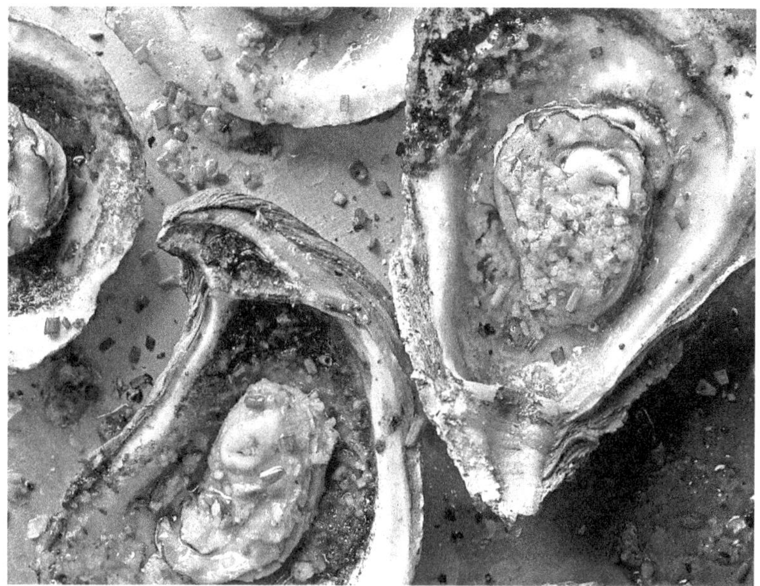

When you are out to impress, there is nothing better than these non-alcoholic grill fired shooters. The juicy and delicious oysters are a great start to any large dinner or outdoor gathering. Just be sure to get more oysters ready because everyone will be after more than one.

Serving Size: 4

Preparation: 5 minutes

Cooking Time: 10 minutes

Ingredients

- 8 x fresh oysters in the shell
- 1/3 cup of fresh lemon juice
- Hot pepper sauce for taste, any brand
- 3 tbsps. of Worcestershire sauce
- Sea salt to taste

Instructions

1. Preheat an outdoor grill to high heat. Assemble **Ingredients** as grill is heating.

2. Carefully add the oysters to the hot grill.

3. Cook for 5 to 10 minutes or until oysters start to open. You can hear the sizzling of juices on the coals when they are ready.

4. Remove your cooked oysters from the grill. Using thick heat resistant gloves or cloth slide a knife between the top and bottom shell to remove the top part.

5. Add to each oyster 2 teaspoons of lemon juice, 1 teaspoon of Worcestershire sauce, then pepper sauce and salt to your liking.

6. Serve the shells while they are still warm.

Traditional Crab Ceviche

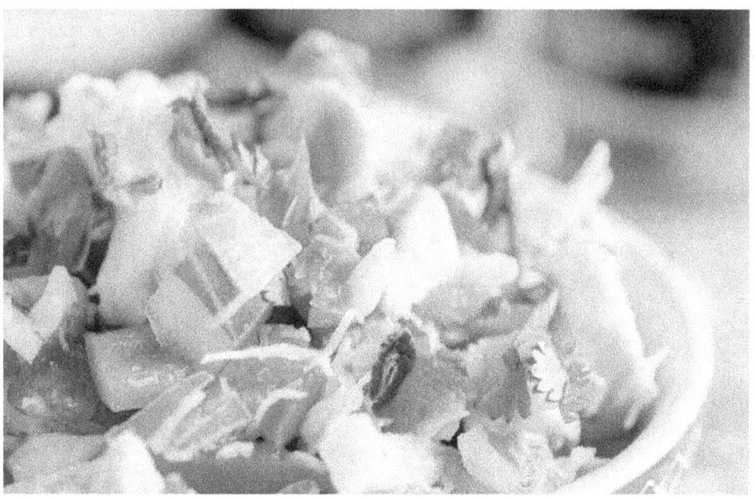

If you are in the mood for something from south of the border, then this easy to make crab ceviche fits the bill nicely. It gets heaps of praise and isn't too heavy on the stomach. It can be eaten with tortillas or with tostadas. Just be sure to make sure it is taken straight from the refrigerator when you are ready to tuck in and eat.

Serving Size: 8

Preparation: 40 minutes

Cooking Time: zero

Ingredients

- 8 oz. pack of imitation crab meat, loosely flake

- 2 x large tomatoes, coarsely chopped

- 1 x large red onion, finely chopped

- 3 x Serrano peppers, removed seeds and finely chop

- 2 limes for the juice

- 1/2 bunch fresh cilantro, roughly chopped

- 1 tbsp. of virgin olive oil

- Salt and black pepper to taste

Instructions

1. Add the flaked (imitation crab) into a glass mixing bowl (can use porcelain). Metal and plastic are not suitable

2. Add and mix the olive oil with the crabmeat until it is well coated. Add and mix the cilantro, chopped onion, chopped tomatoes, and the serrano peppers

3. Once mixed, squeeze lime juice to cover everything. Mix well

4. Season liberally with sea salt and black pepper

5. Refrigerate for around one hour before ready to serve

Burgundy Wine Cooked Mushrooms

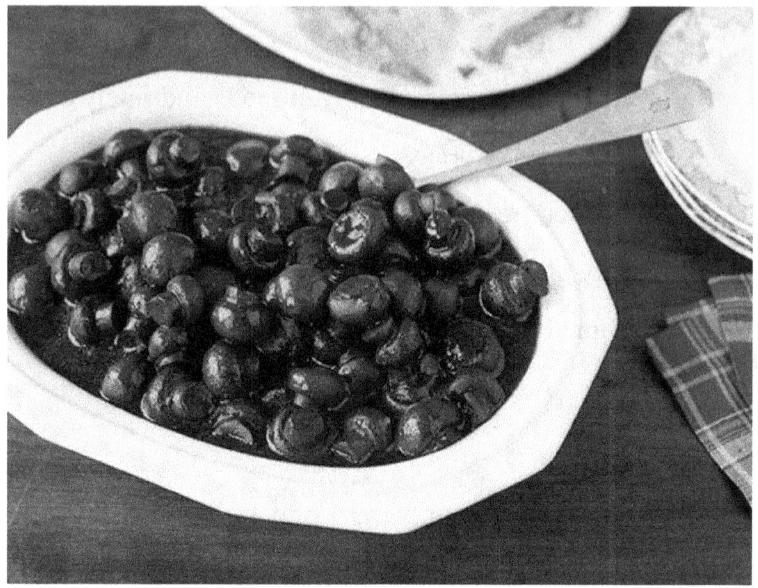

These may be in the appetizer section, but they make a fantastic side dish to accompany any meat dish you may have. The thick broth and red wine are super tasty, and the mushrooms are super succulent. Try with thin strips of beef, and you will soon have a weekly favorite.

Serving Size: 4

Preparation: 10 minutes

Cooking Time: 30 minutes

Ingredients

- 1 x large onion, diced
- 1 x 10.5 oz. can of beef broth
- 2 x 8 oz. cans of whole mushrooms, drained and reserve liquid from one of the cans
- 1/3 cup of Red Burgundy wine

Instructions

1. Place a small pan over medium heat. Add the beef broth and onion and simmer for 15 minutes

2. Add the mushrooms and the canned liquid

3. Add the wine and continue to simmer until the liquid reduces by half, around 15 minutes

4. Serve warm with rest of meal

Speedy Baked Zucchini Chips

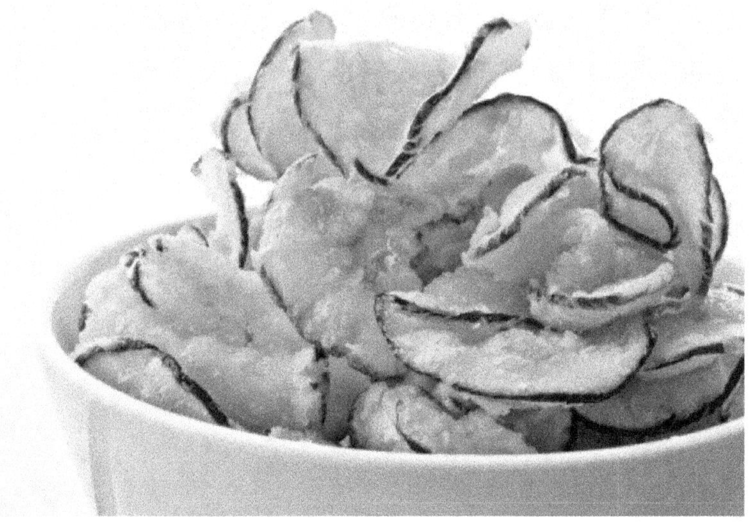

If you want to play sneaky with the kids and get them to eat something healthy from the garden, then this can be just the thing. With the seasoned breadcrumbs, they won't have any idea they are munching on some homegrown goodness. Have them as a nightly snack or make a few to get everyone in a healthy mood.

Serving Size: 4

Preparation: 5 minutes

Cooking Time: 10 minutes

Ingredients

- 2 zucchini medium-sized. Cut 1/4-inch thick slices
- 1/2 cup of dry bread crumbs, seasoned
- 1/8 tsp. of fresh ground black pepper
- 2 x tbsps. of Parmesan cheese, grated
- 2 x large egg whites

Instructions

1. Preheat the oven to 475 degrees Fahrenheit. Grease a none stick baking sheet

2. Add the breadcrumbs, black pepper, and the Parmesan cheese, mix to combine

3. Add the egg whites to another bowl and whisk gently

4. Take each zucchini slice and dip in the egg whites. Dredge through the breadcrumb mix.

5. Place onto the baking sheet

6. Bake for 5 minutes. Turn over then bake for an additional 5 or 10 minutes until they brown and crisp

Mango Salsa

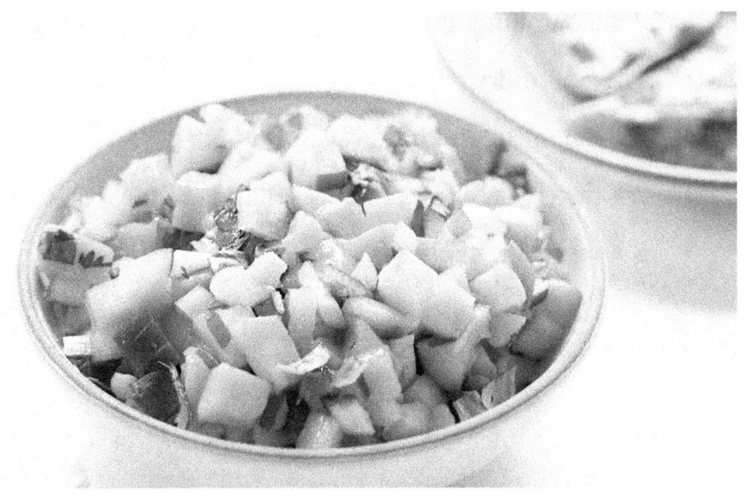

Break out the blackened fish recipes because they go great with this salsa. Either that or whip some up for a tasty dip with tortillas or another healthy dipping food. If you are trying to combat your cholesterol, anyone would think you were not telling the truth after they taste this dish.

Serving Size: 8

Preparation: 15 minutes

Cooking Time: 0 minutes

Ingredients

- 1 large mango, peel, remove seed and roughly chop
- 1 x large red pepper, remove seeds and finely chop
- 1 x green onion, roughly chopped
- 1 x jalapeno pepper, chopped finely
- 2 tbsps. of fresh cilantro coarsely chop
- 2 tbsps. of limejuice
- 1 tbsp. of lemon juice

Instructions

1. Add to a medium mixing bowl the mix mango, chopped bell pepper, onion, jalapeno the cilantro and lemon and lime juice

2. Gently mix

3. Cover the bowl and set aside for around 30 minutes before you are ready to serve

Main Dishes

Nikujaga Japanese-styled Comfort Food

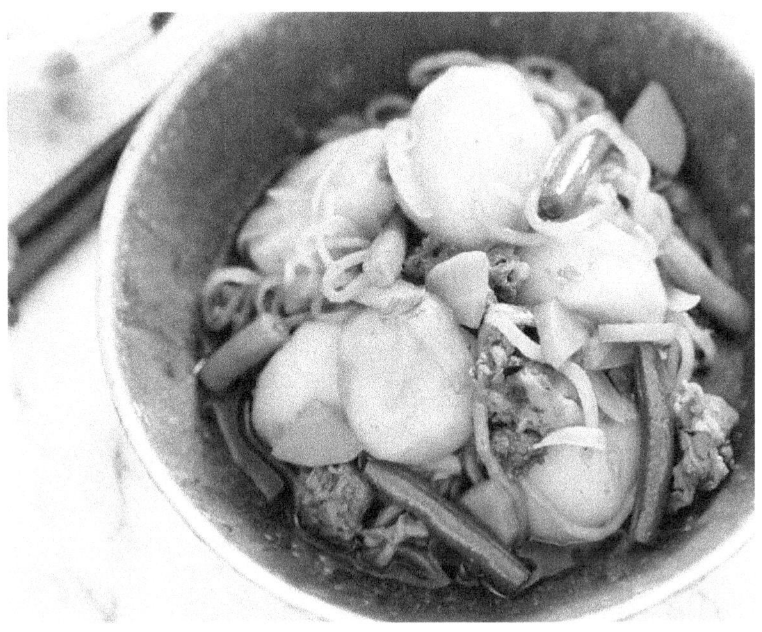

This is one of the top comfort foods in Japan. Thinly sliced beef cooked with tender potatoes and onions. These are perfect to accompany shirataki noodles. For something different on a cold night in the fall, then this is perfect for warming and satisfying the belly.

Serving Size: 4

Preparation: 15 minutes

Cooking Time: 35 minutes

Ingredients

- 1/4 lb. of sirloin steak, thinly sliced
- 4 x large potatoes, cut into mouth-sized pieces
- 1 x large onion, coarsely chopped
- 1/2 cup of snow peas
- 1 tbsp. of vegetable oil
- 2 cups of dashi soup
- 1/4 cup of soy sauce
- 1/4 cup of Japanese Sake
- 1 tbsp. of white sugar

Instructions

1. Add the snow peas into a small pan and cover with water

2. Bring to a rolling boil and then remove from heat. Drain well and set on one side

3. Place a large skillet on medium-high heat and add the oil

4. Add the beef and cook until browned.

5. Carefully add the potatoes. Cook for 5 to 7 minutes or until soft

6. Add in the dashi soup, sake, soy sauce, and the sugar to the mixture. Simmer on medium for 10 minutes

7. Reduce to low and sprinkle the onion on the top of the mix. Continue simmering for 15 minutes until most of the liquid has evaporated

8. Add the snow peas when ready to serve

Easy Italian Fagioli

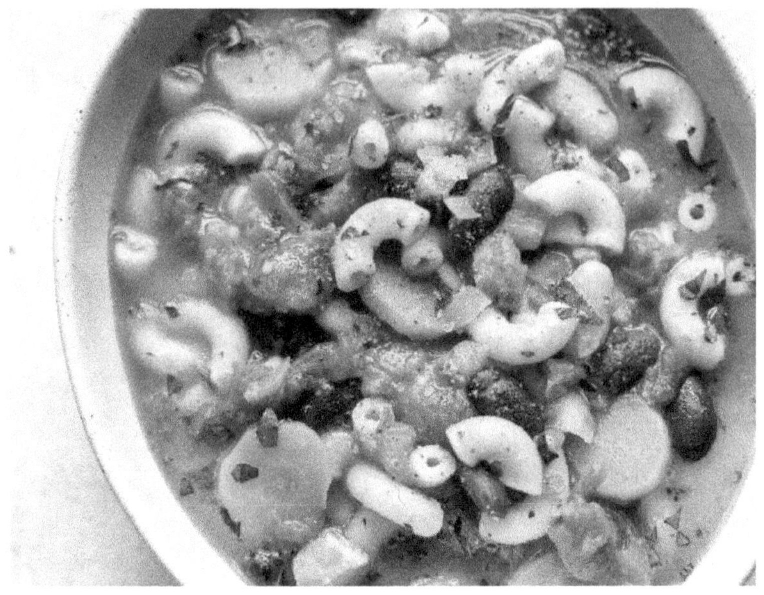

Here is a great Italian styled pasta dish that will warm the coldest family member. Taking hardly any effort and just 30 minutes to cook, it can be eaten for lunch or a heartwarming dinner after a day outside. Just be careful to leave enough space for a healthy dessert.

Serving Size: 4

Preparation: 10 minutes

Cooking Time: 30 minutes

Ingredients

- 1 1/2 cups of Ditalini pasta
- 1 x 15 oz. can of cannellini beans, drain and rinse
- 1 x 14 oz. can of chicken broth
- 4 x 8 oz. cans of tomato sauce
- 1 tbsp. of virgin olive oil
- 1 large carrot, diced small
- 1 large stalk of celery, diced small
- 1 small onion, finely diced
- 2 garlic cloves, chopped finely
- Ground black pepper for taste
- 1 tbsp. of dried parsley
- 1/2 tbsp. of dried basil leaves

Instructions

1. On medium to high heat, add and heat the oil in a large saucepan. Add the carrot, onion, and celery and sauté until soft. Add the garlic to sauté for a couple of minutes

2. Add the broth, tomato sauce, pepper, basil, and parsley. Continue to simmer for a further 20 minutes

3. In a large pot boil some salted water. Add the Ditalini pasta. Cook until al dente or 8 minutes then drain

4. Add the can of beans to the mixture. Simmer for a few minutes until heated through

5. Once pasta cooks, add into the sauce and bean mixture

6. Serve immediately

Grilled Salmon with Cilantro

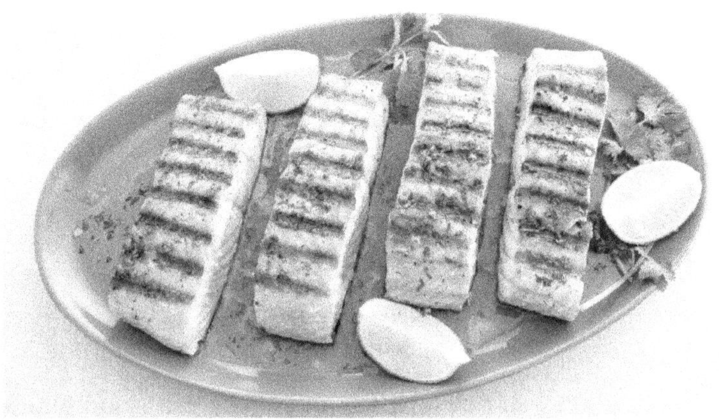

When you are in the yard, and the grill is getting hot, there is nothing better you can cook that will impress everyone. Delicious marinated salmon is succulent where all the flavors of cilantro, garlic, honey, and zesty lime burst all the taste buds in the mouth. Time in the garden never felt so rewarding.

Serving Size: 6

Preparation: 15 minutes

Cooking Time: 20 m

Ingredients

- 4 salmon steaks

- 2 x cups of honey
- 1 bunch fresh cilantro leaves, finely chopped
- 2 x garlic cloves, finely chopped
- 1 x large lime for juice
- Salt and black pepper to taste

Instructions

1. Take a small saucepan and place it on low-medium heat. Add the cilantro, honey, garlic, and lime juice, stir while cooking

2. Heat for 5-minutes until the honey mixes easy

3. Remove the pan from the heat, and let cool a little

4. In a baking dish, add the salmon steaks and season well with sea salt and black pepper. Cover the salmon with the marinade. Cover and refrigerate for 10 minutes

5. Bring an outdoor grill to high heat

6. Oil the grill grate lightly. Add the salmon steaks and cook until the fish flakes or for around 5 minutes.

7. Serve while warm

Italian Porcini Mushroom Pasta

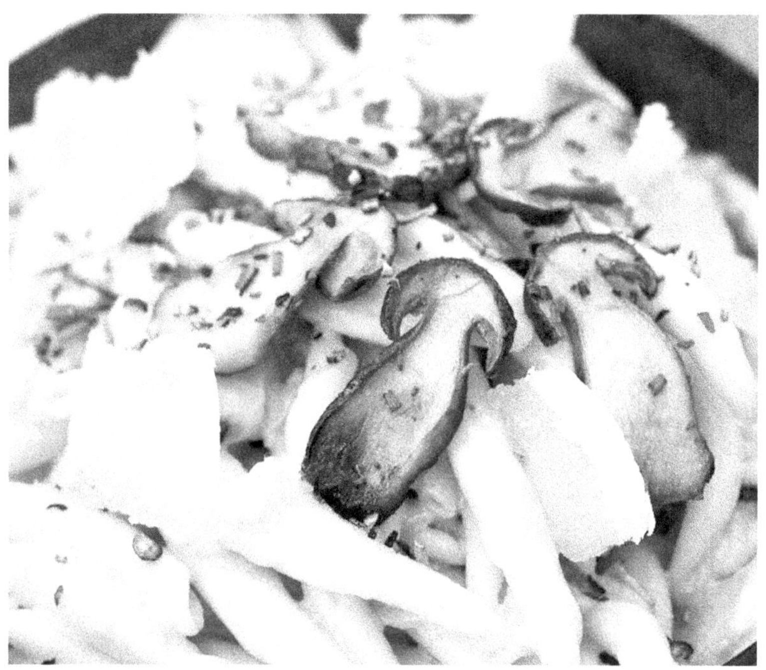

This dish is perfect because you can use any pasta you have lying around. However, wide flat pasta takes this to another level. The thick and tasty mushroom sauce is a delight as you taste all the herbs, the red wine, and the thick creamy sauce that makes you want more and more.

Serving Size: 6

Preparation: 10 minutes

Cooking Time: 18 minutes

Ingredients

- 6 cups of Tagliatelle / Fettucine or other wide noodles
- 1 cup of porcini mushrooms, rehydrated
- 1 1/2 cups of tomatoes, crushed
- 1 x large red bell pepper, remove seeds and julienne
- 1 medium carrot, julienne
- 1/2 cup of dry red wine
- 1/2 large red onion, minced
- 2 x garlic cloves, minced
- 1 tbsp. of virgin olive oil
- 2 tsp. of fresh basil, coarsely chopped
- 1 tsp. of dried rosemary, crushed
- Sea salt and ground black pepper for taste

Instructions

1. Place a large skillet over medium-high heat and warm the olive oil

2. Add the garlic and minced onions. Sauté for around 4 minutes

3. Add the bell pepper, and carrots then sauté for another 4 minutes

4. Add the wine and raise the heat. Boil for 1-minute

5. Reduce the heat to medium-low. Add in the mushrooms and cook for a further 3 minutes

6. Add in the tomatoes, the basil, and the rosemary. Season with sea salt and fresh ground black pepper

7. Simmer for around 10 minutes then serve immediately over cooked noodles

Pulled Slow-Cooker Pork

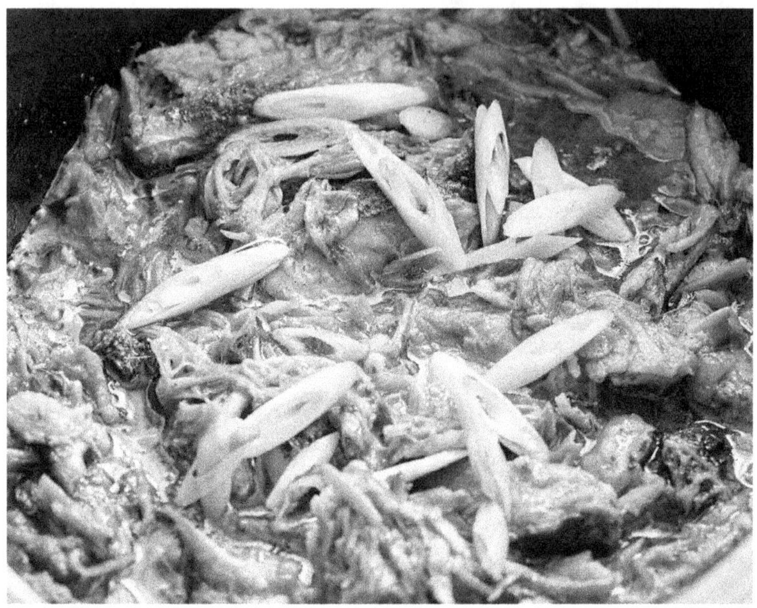

This pork is cooked to perfection when you use a slow cooker. It just flakes in the mouth. The root beer adds another dimension you don't find with other dishes. Add in some of your favorite BBQ flavored sauce, and you are in for a belly-busting treat as you munch through the thick tasty burger buns filled with succulent delights.

Serving Size: 8

Preparation: 10 minutes

Cooking Time: 7 hours

Ingredients

- 2 lb. of pork tenderloin
- 1 x 12 fluid oz. can/bottle of root beer
- 1 x 18 oz. bottle of barbecue sauce desired flavor
- 8 x hamburger buns, cut in half and toast lightly

Instructions

1. In your slow cooker, add the pork tenderloin. Cover with the root beer

2. Place on the lid then on low cook for 6 - 7 hours until you can shred the pork.

3. Note: Cooking times can vary according to differences your slow cooker.

4. Drain well. Stir in the barbecue sauce and mix with the pork.

5. Add to the hamburger buns and serve immediately

Homemade Black Bean Veggie Burgers

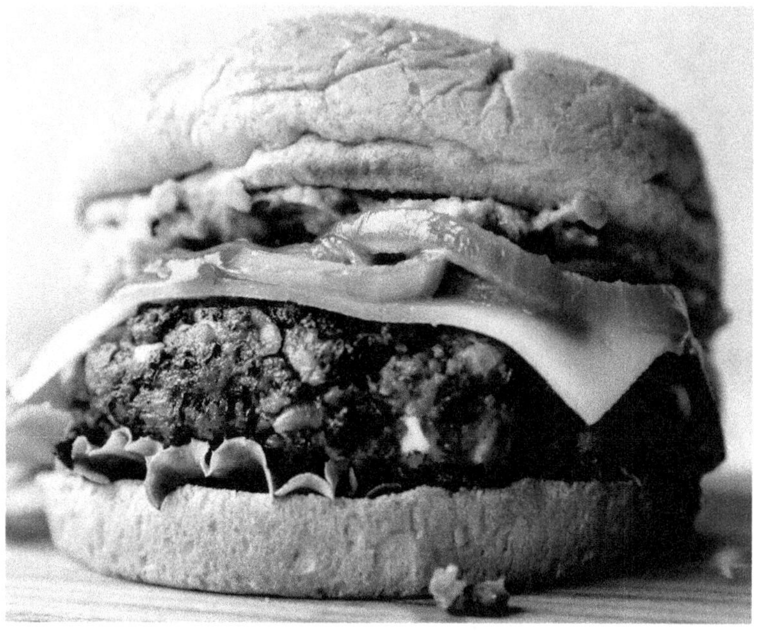

If you struggle to get the kids to eat veggies, or you are fed up with those frozen veggie burgers, then these can fit the bill. With a little hint of spice and the texture of the black beans, these will soon be a firm favorite around the home. Add a bit more hot sauce and a bit of salad, and you will be looking forward to burgers on any night of the week.

Serving Size: 4

Preparation: 15 minutes

Cooking Time: 20 minutes

Ingredients

- 1 x 16 oz. can of black beans, drain and rinse
- 1/2 large green bell pepper, remove seeds and slice into 2-inch pieces
- 1/2 large onion, cut into wedge shapes
- 3 x garlic cloves
- 1 large egg
- 1 tbsp. of chili powder
- 1 tbsp. of ground cumin
- 1 tsp. of hot sauce or Thai chili sauce
- 1/2 cup of seasoned breadcrumbs

Instructions

1. Option 1: If using an outdoor grill, preheat the grill to high heat. Oil a sheet of aluminum foil lightly

2. Option 2: If using an oven. Preheat the oven to 375 degrees Fahrenheit. Oil a baking sheet lightly

3. In a medium mixing bowl, add the black beans. Smash with a fork until you have a thick consistency

4. Add the Bell pepper, onion, and garlic to a food processor. Chop and then stir into the smashed black beans

5. In a small mixing bowl, add the egg, chili sauce, chili powder, and cumin. Mix well

6. Add the egg mix to the beans. Add in the breadcrumbs and mix until the mixture holds together.

7. Split and make into four patties

8. When grilling, place each of the patties on the foil. Grill for around 8 minutes on both sides.

9. When baking, place the patties onto the baking sheet. Bake for around 10 minutes on both sides

Red and Spicy Lentil Curry

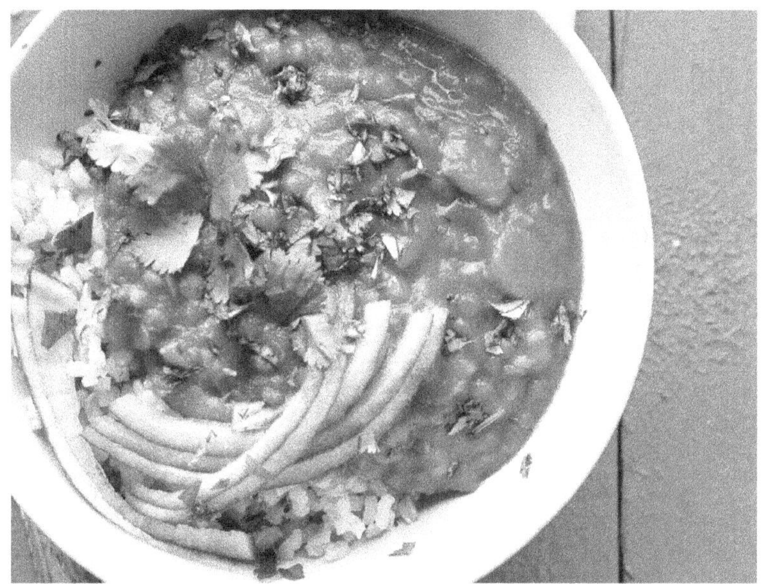

You can use this as a side dish or a bit of a dip for naan bread. Nevertheless, this spicy red lentil curry is perfect on its own with rice or anything else you feel like serving it with. It is easy to prepare and will take as long as a steaming hot pan full of fresh basmati rice.

A few Indian flavors can make any meal that little more exotic.

Serving Size: 8

Preparation: 10 minutes

Cooking Time: 30 minutes

Ingredients

- 2 cups of red lentils
- 1 x 14.25 oz. can of tomato puree
- 1 large onion, diced roughly
- 2 tbsps. of curry paste
- 1 tbsp. of curry powder
- 1 tsp. of garlic, minced
- 1 tsp. of fresh ginger, minced
- 1 tsp. of ground turmeric
- 1 tsp. of ground cumin
- 1 tsp. of chili powder
- 1 tsp. of white sugar
- 1 tbsp. of vegetable oil
- 1 tsp. of salt

Instructions

1. Rinse the lentils with cold water until it runs clear.

2. Add the lentils into a large pot. Cover with water. Bring to a rolling boil and cover

3. Reduce the heat to medium-low and simmer for 15 to 20 minutes. Add more water as needed while cooking. Drain when lentils are tender

4. Place a large skillet over medium-high heat. Heat the oil, add the onions and cook for around 20 minutes until caramelized

5. In a large bowl, combine the curry paste, the curry powder, cumin, chili powder, turmeric, salt, ginger, sugar, and garlic. Mix and then add to the onions

6. Raise heat to high. Cook for 1 or 2 minutes until fragrant, stir to avoid burning

7. Add the tomato puree and heat through. Remove from the heat then add to the lentils and mix.

8. Serve hot.

Thick and Chewy Dumplings

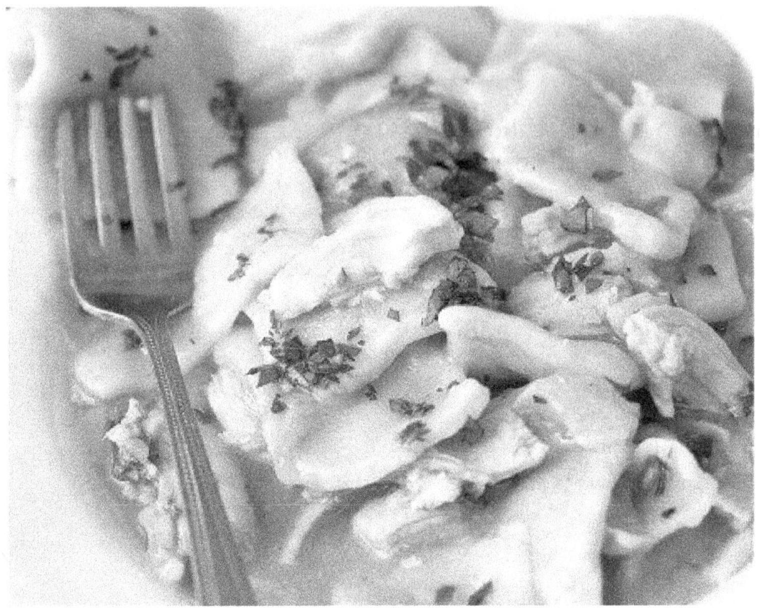

These dumplings are fantastic when dropped in soups or stews. They can quickly transform a meal into something that satisfies and fills every member of the family after a day out. To boost any everyday dish, these can make a nice change to potatoes or bread.

Serving Size: 6

Preparation: 5 minutes

Cooking Time: 15 minutes

Ingredients

- 1 cup of flour, all-purpose and sifted
- 2 tsp. of baking-powder
- 1 tbsp. of butter
- 1/2 cup of fresh milk
- 1 tsp. of white granulated sugar
- 1/2 tsp. of salt

Instructions

1. In a medium mixing bowl, add the flour, salt, sugar and baking powder. Cut in the butter and mix until it forms a crumbly mixture.

2. Add the milk and stir to form a soft dough.

3. Add spoonful's into soup or boiling stew.

4. Cover and continue to simmer for around 15 minutes. Don't lift the lid.

5. Serve hot

Spring Onions with Mongolian Beef

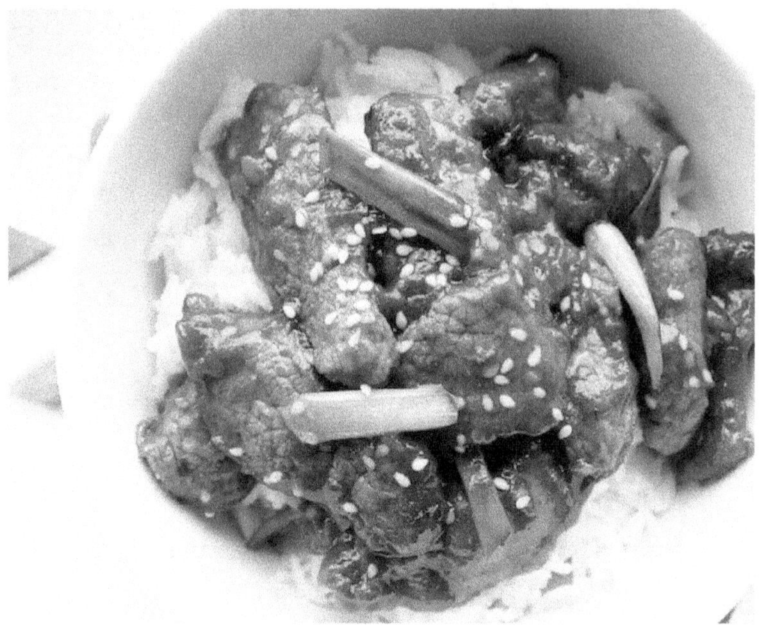

This soy-based sweet and sticky Chinese dish is a delight with soft noodles or a plate full of healthy rice. It takes hardly any time to cook and is a delight to add something very different to the dinner table. The hint of garlic and ginger brings a sense of the orient with this new family favorite.

Serving Size: 4

Preparation: 12 minutes

Cooking Time: 8 minutes

Ingredients

- 1 lb. of beef flank steak, slice into 1/4 inch diagonal strips
- 1 cup of vegetable oil to deep fry
- 2/3 cup of dark brown granulated sugar
- 1/2 tsp. of fresh ginger, grated
- 1/2 cup of soy sauce
- 2 garlic cloves, finely chopped
- 2 tsp. of vegetable oil
- 1/2 cup of plain water
- 1/4 cup of cornstarch
- 2 bunches fresh green onions, sliced in 2-inch lengths

Instructions

1. Place a saucepan over medium-high heat. Heat the vegetable oil and add the garlic and ginger. Cook while stirring for around 30 seconds until fragrant

2. Add the water, soy sauce, and the brown sugar

3. Increase the heat to medium to high. Stir until the sugar dissolves in about 4 minutes. The sauce should thicken slightly

4. Remove from the heat, and set on one side

5. In a mixing bowl, add the beef and cover with the cornstarch, mix until well coated.

6. Let the beef and cornstarch mix sit for around 10 minutes until almost most of the meat juices have been absorbed

7. In a deep skillet, heat the vegetable oil to 375 degrees F

8. Shake off any excess cornstarch from the beef. Carefully add to the hot oil

9. Cook for around 2-minutes until the edges crisp and brown

10. Using a slotted spoon remove from the oil. Drain on paper towels

11. Remove the oil from the skillet then return to the heat

12. Add the meat back to the pan. Stir briefly and add the reserved sugar mixture

13. Stir gently then add the onions

14. Bring back to a boil. Cook for around 2-minutes till the onions soften and are bright green

15. Serve warm

Authentic Amatriciana

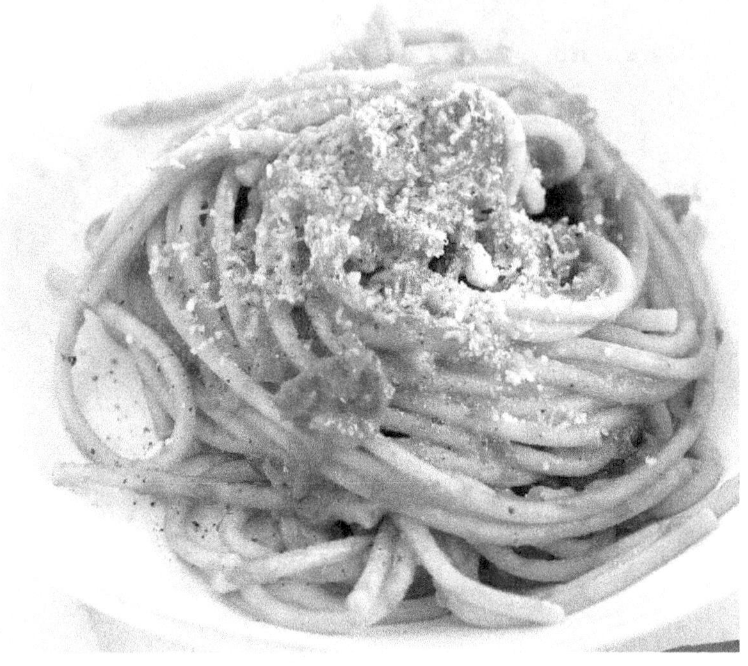

Eating Italian is as healthy as anything is, and this authentic Amatriciana dish is no different. The sweetness of the tomatoes blends with the bacon strips, and the slight hint of spice from the pepper flakes. A healthy dose of pasta and topped with parmesan makes this a super cholesterol-lowering favorite.

Serving Size: 4

Preparation: 15 minutes

Cooking Time: 20 minutes

Ingredients

- 4 slices bacon, cut into small squares
- 1 lb. of linguine pasta, uncooked. Can use other flat pasta as an alternative
- 2 x 14.5 oz. can of stewed tomatoes
- 1 medium onion, coarsely chopped, about 1/2 cup
- 1 tsp. of garlic, minced
- 1/4 tsp. of red pepper flakes
- 1 tbsp. of fresh basil, coarsely chopped
- 2 tbsps. of Parmesan cheese, grated

Instructions

1. Place a large skillet over medium to high heat. Cook the diced bacon for around 5 minutes until crispy. Drain all the dripping apart from about 2 tablespoons from the pan

2. Add the onions and cook for 3 minutes on medium heat. Add garlic, and red pepper flakes then cook for 30 seconds until fragrant

3. Add the cans of tomatoes with juice. Simmer for 10 minutes while breaking the tomatoes

4. In a large pot of lightly salted water. Cook the pasta until al dente and drain well

5. Add the basil into the tomato sauce. Stir and toss in with the cooked pasta

6. Serve hot with grated Parmesan cheese on top

Secret Spiced Blackened Tilapia

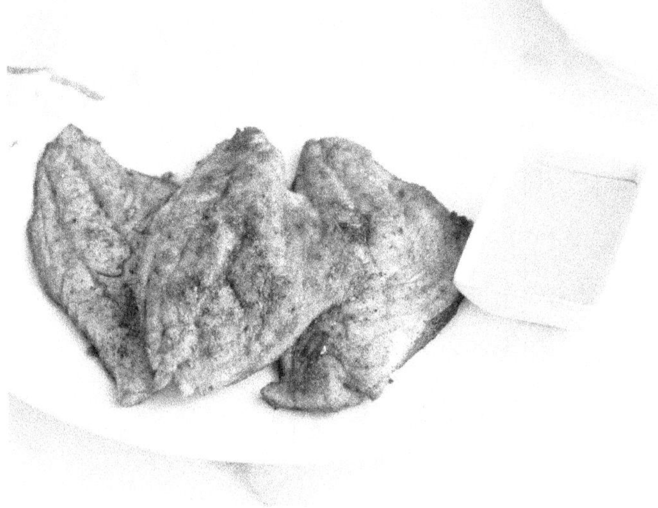

Sometimes recipes crop up unexpectedly. This secret spice for this blackened fish dish transforms it into something very unexpected. The paprika delivers a little hint of sweetness while the cayenne delivers that all-important kick. Heat the skillet and watch as all the spices blacken to give that grill-charred appearance.

Serving Size: 4

Preparation: 10 minutes

Cooking Time: 8 minutes

Ingredients

- 1 lb. of fresh tilapia fillets
- 1 medium lemon, cut into wedges
- 4 large slices white bread
- 3 tbsps. of paprika
- 1 tbsp. of onion powder
- 1 pinch of garlic powder
- 1 tsp. of cayenne pepper, or to desired taste
- 1 tsp. of dried oregano, crushed
- 1 tsp. of dried thyme, crushed
- 1/2 tsp. of celery seed
- 1 tsp. of ground white pepper
- 1 tsp. of ground black pepper
- 1 tbsp. of Sea salt, or to taste
- 1 tbsp. of vegetable oil

Instructions

1. Take a small jar or plastic container with a lid. Add the paprika, garlic powder, onion powder, white and black pepper, cayenne, celery, thyme, oregano, and salt. Close the lid and shake to mix

2. Cover the fish fillets all over with the spices and set aside at room temperature for 30 minutes maximum

3. Place a heavy skillet over high heat. Add the oil and heat till nearly smoking

4. Place the fish in the pan. Cook for until the fish is opaque, around 3 minutes on either side. It should flake easily with a fork

5. Remove fillets from the skillet. Place onto white bread slices

6. Drizzle the juices from the pan then squeeze lemon juice across the top

7. Note: all the juices will soak into the bread

Mexican Quinoa One Skillet Recipe

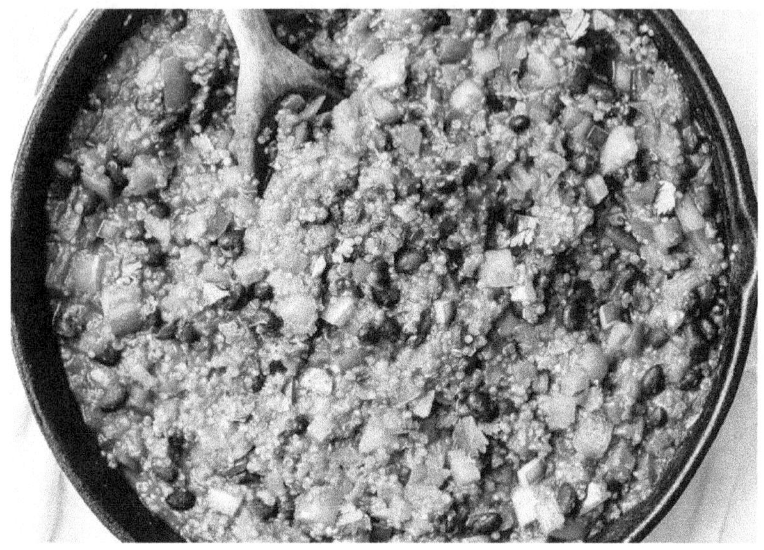

From one of the world, healthiest foods come one of the healthiest dishes you could wish for. This superfood skillet recipe delivers a healthy dose of quinoa, the sweet taste of corn, and the salty bite of black beans. Add in some creamy avocado and the fiery kick of chili flakes and the chopped jalapeno, and you have a dish like nothing else you will have ever tasted.

Serving Size: 4

Preparation: 15 minutes

Cooking Time: 25 minutes

Ingredients

- 1 cup of quinoa
- 1 cup of yellow corn
- 1 x 15 oz. can of black beans, rinse and drain
- 1 x 14.5 oz. can of diced tomatoes, fire-roasted
- 1 large avocado, peel, remove seed and dice
- 1 jalapeno pepper, remove seeds and chop
- 1 cup of chicken broth
- 2 x garlic cloves, cut or mince
- 1 tbsp. of virgin olive oil
- 1 tbsp. of red pepper flakes, or to taste
- 1 1/2 tsp. of chili powder
- 1/2 tsp. of cumin
- 1 x pinch sea salt and fresh ground black pepper to taste
- 1 medium lime for juice
- 2 tbsps. of fresh cilantro coarsely chopped

Instructions

1. Put a large skillet over medium-high heat and add the oil. Sauté the jalapeno's and garlic for around one minute until fragrant.

2. Add in the black beans, corn, quinoa, tomatoes, and chicken broth. Stir as it simmers and add the chili powder, pepper flakes, and the cumin. Season with salt and black pepper add more spices if required.

3. Adjust the heat to medium low and simmer. Cover and cook for around 20 minutes until the quinoa becomes soft and tender. Most of the liquid should be absorbed.

4. When cooked, stir in the avocado, lime juice, and cilantro.

Vegetarian Un-Sloppy Joes

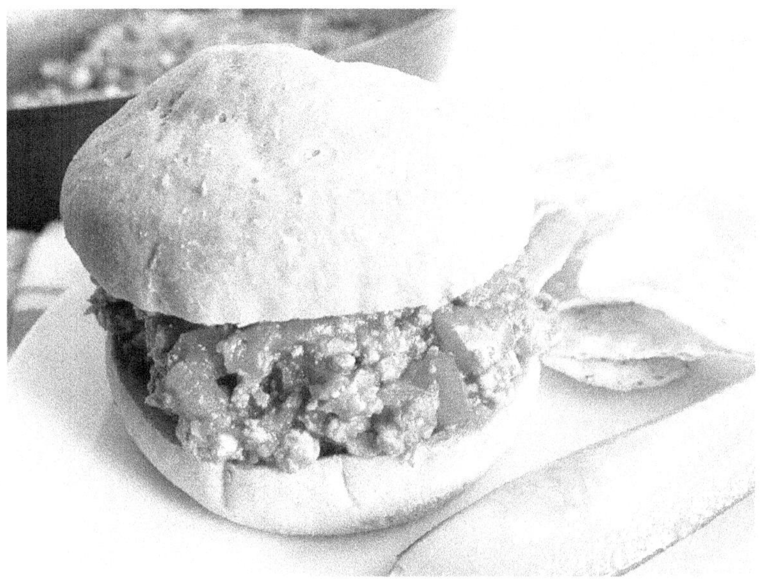

These Joes can't be guaranteed not to be sloppy, but they will be guaranteed to be tasty and so much fun to eat. Munch through the Kaiser bun to find the spiced up vegetarian mulch that makes up the filling of this sandwich. They may not contain any meat, yet not one person will complain as they tackle the Joe that sits in front of them.

Serving Size: 8

Preparation: 15 minutes

Cooking Time: 15 minutes

Ingredients

- 8 large Kaiser rolls
- 1 x 14.5 oz. can of diced tomatoes
- 1 x 15 oz. can of kidney beans, rinse and drain well
- 1/2 cup of chopped onion
- 1/2 cup of chopped celery
- 1/2 cup of chopped carrots
- 1 tbsp. of virgin olive oil
- 1 green bell pepper, remove seeds and cut
- 2 x garlic cloves, minced
- 1 1/2 tbsps. of chili powder
- 1 tbsp. of tomato paste
- 1 tbsp. of distilled white vinegar
- 1 tsp. of fresh ground black pepper

Instructions

1. Over medium heat, place a skillet, and add the oil.

2. Add the onion, carrot, celery, peppers, and garlic. Sauté until they are all tender.

3. Add the tomatoes, tomato paste, chili powder, vinegar, and the pepper. Reduce and simmer with the skillet covered for 10 minutes.

4. Add the kidney beans; cook while stirring for a further 5 minutes.

5. Slice a 1/4 inch from the top of the Kaiser rolls and set aside. Scoop out the center of the rolls and leave about 1/2 inch to form a thick shell. Keep the inside of rolls to be sued for breadcrumbs or other uses.

6. Spoon sloppy bean mixture into roll hollows and top with the bread slice

7. Serve immediately.

Pasta Mexicana

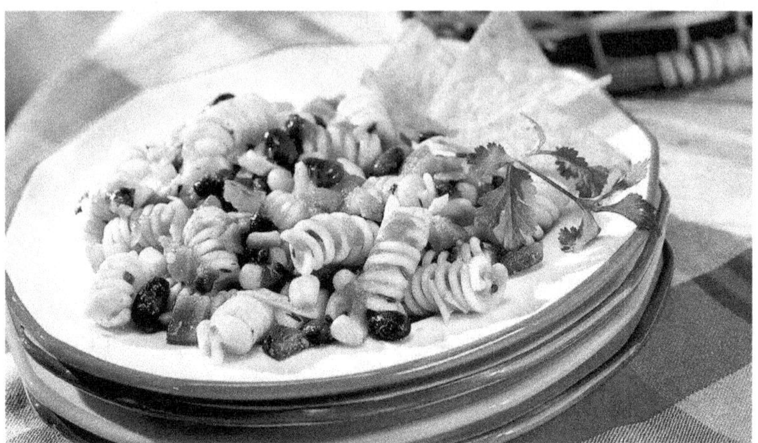

This dish is worthy of Speedy Gonzalez himself. It takes a few minutes to cook, but anyone who samples it will think it has taken ages; there is so much southern flavor. Salty black beans, with chopped olives on slightly al dente pasta. For something you can make in fifteen minutes, this is fantastic for a quick lunch or a light dinner before putting your feet up.

Serving Size: 4

Preparation: 5 minutes

Cooking Time: 15 minutes

Ingredients

- 1/2 lb. of shell pasta
- 1/2 cup of sweet corn kernels
- 1 15 oz. can of black beans, rinse and drain well
- 1 14.5 oz. can of peeled, diced tomatoes
- 2 medium onions, roughly chopped
- 1 green bell pepper, remove seeds and cut
- 1 1/2 tbsps. of taco seasoning mix
- 2 tbsps. of virgin olive oil
- 1/4 cup of salsa
- 1/4 cup of sliced black olives
- Sea salt and black pepper for taste

Instructions

1. Boil a large lightly salted pot of water. Insert your pasta and cook until it feels al dente, around 8 or 10 minutes. Be sure to drain well.

2. As the pasta cooks, place a large skillet on medium to high heat. Add some olive oil and sauté the onions and pepper until browned for around 10 minutes.

3. Add the corn to heat through. Add the tomatoes, salsa, black beans, olives, and the taco seasoning — season with salt and black pepper. Cook while stirring for around 5 minutes until heated through.

4. Take the pasta and toss it with the sauce mixture.

5. Serve hot.

Speedy Tuna Casserole

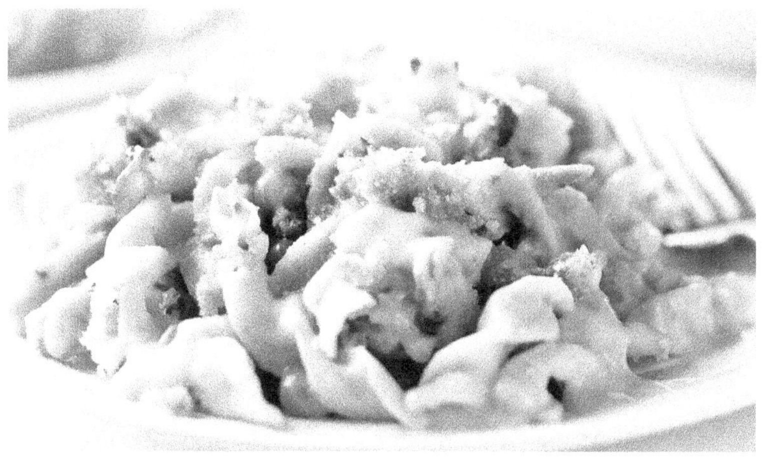

Here you have one of the tastiest casseroles ever using canned tuna. It doesn't take long to prepare or cook, but it is one-hundred percent satisfying for everyone who sits around the dinner table. It may have a pack of dried macaroni and cheese, but it is one healthy dish for anyone who is trying to lower their cholesterol.

Serving Size: 4

Preparation: 5 minutes

Cooking Time: 20 minutes

Ingredients

- 1 x 10.75 oz. can of condensed cream of mushroom soup
- 1 x 9 oz. can of tuna, drained
- 1 x 10 oz. can of can peas, drained
- 1 x7.25 oz. pack of macaroni and cheese mix

Instructions

1. Take the macaroni and cheese mix. Prepare according to directions on the package.

2. Once ready, add in the cream of mushroom soup, canned tuna, and peas.

3. Mix to combine then heat until it begins to bubble.

Cuban Sweet and Spicy Black Beans

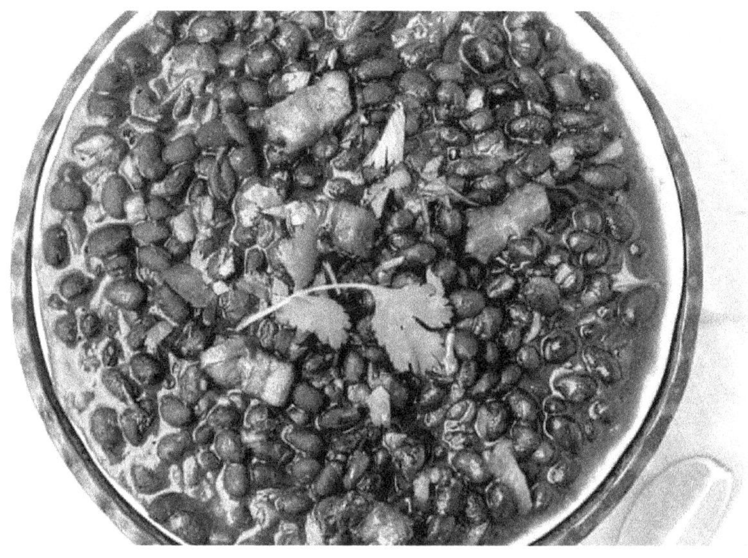

Anyone who has ever tasted Cuban beans will love these. A little sweet and a little spicy is the perfect combination. It makes a change from the regular red beans in chili to swap them for lashings of black beans. These are a fantastic alternative to other dishes to serve over rice or even spooned over a large serving of fries.

Serving Size: 8

Preparation: 15 minutes

Cooking Time: 90 minutes

Ingredients

- 1 lb. of black beans, wash and drain
- 1 large green onion, roughly chopped
- 1 x 6 oz. can of tomato paste
- 1 x 4 oz. jar of diced pimentos drained well
- 1 large green bell pepper, chop roughly
- 1/4 cup of virgin olive oil
- 6 x garlic cloves, minced
- 5 cups of water
- 1 tbsp. of vinegar
- 2 tsps. of sea salt
- 1 tsp. of white sugar
- 1 tsp. of ground black pepper

Instructions

1. Put the beans in a large container and cover with water. Soak for at least 8-hours, overnight preferable. Drain and rinse before use.

2. Place a medium-sized pan on medium heat. Add the oil and heat. Sauté the onion, peppers, and minced garlic until soft and fragrant.

3. Add in the water, beans, pimentos, tomato paste, and the vinegar.

4. Stir and then season with sea salt, black pepper, and sugar.

5. Raise the heat and bring up to boil. Reduce heat, so it simmers and then cover the saucepan.

6. Simmer for 1-1/2 hours and stir occasionally. Beans should finally be tender.

7. Serve with rice.

Spiced Indian Dahl

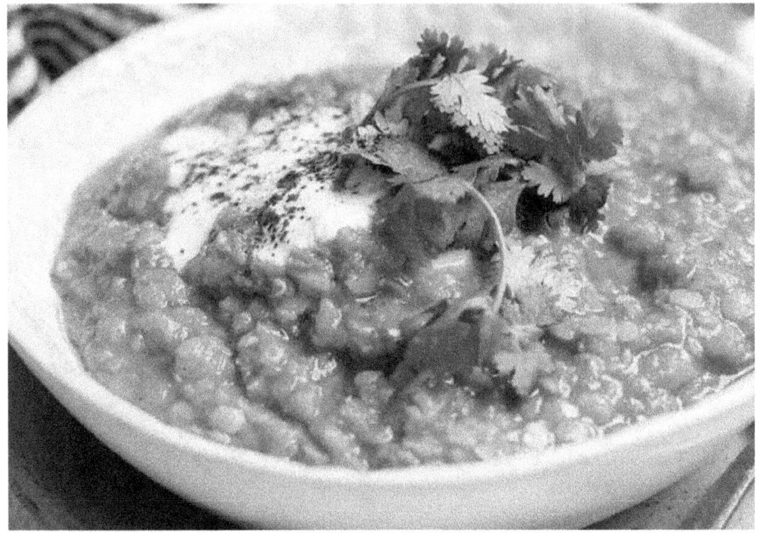

If you are after a flexible dish, then this Indian Dahl might be the one. You can make it a bit more soup-like to dip your naan or make it regular and spoon it over rice. Either way, it is a taste of India that can warm any stomach.

Serving Size: 6

Preparation: 15 minutes

Cooking Time: 40 minutes

Ingredients

- 1 cup of red lentils
- 4 large tomatoes, coarsely chopped
- 3 medium jalapeno peppers, remove seeds and mince
- 3 medium onions, coarsely chopped
- 6 x garlic cloves, minced
- 2 tbsps. of ginger, minced
- 1 tsp. of mustard seed
- 2 tbsps. of fresh cilantro, coarsely chopped
- 1 tbsp. of ground cumin
- 1 tbsp. of ground coriander seed
- 2 tbsps. of virgin olive oil
- 1 cup of water
- Sea salt to taste

Instructions

1. Add the lentils to a saucepan or pressure cooker with water to cover. Cook until soft. Pressure cookers are faster at doing this.

2. Heat a large skillet on medium-high heat. Add the oil and then the mustard seeds. As the seeds start to flutter, add in

the onions, garlic, jalapeno, and ginger. Sauté until fragrant, and the onions and garlic begin to become golden brown.

3. Add the chopped tomatoes, cumin, and coriander. Simmer until the tomatoes are cooked well.

4. Add the water and bring to a boil for 6 minutes.

5. Add in the cooked lentils. Stir well and add salt for taste.

6. Remove from heat and add the chopped cilantro.

7. Serve immediately.

Tasty and Spicy Beef Stir-Fry

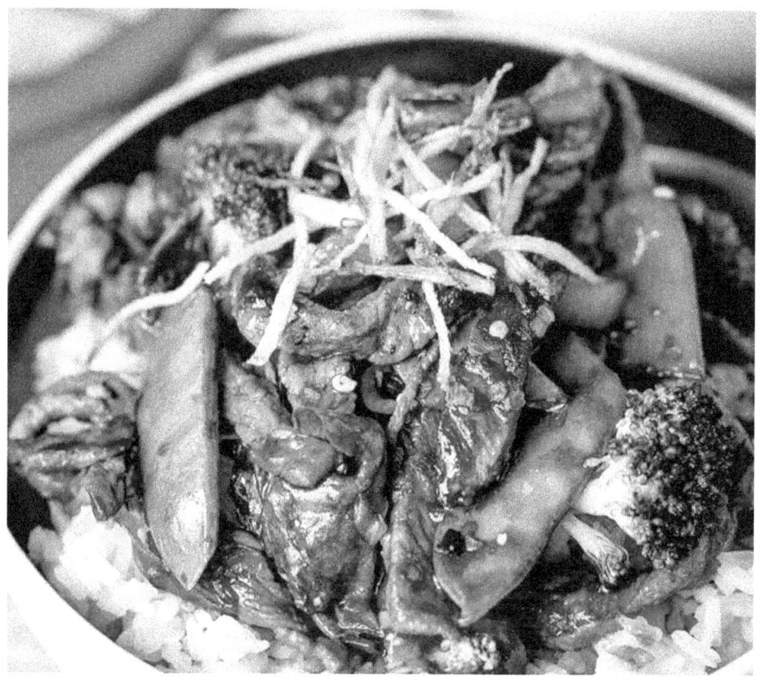

There aren't many dishes that are as tasty and as healthy as a traditional stir-fry. While using minimal spices, this beef dish has tons of flavor and plenty of crunchy, healthy veggies. It is easy to make after a bit of preparation, and it is one dish that, when served with rice, can satisfy and Chinese dish fan.

Serving Size: 4

Preparation: 10 minutes

Cooking Time: 60 minutes

Ingredients

- 2 cups of brown rice
- 1 lb. of boneless beef round steak, cut into thin strips
- 3 cups of broccoli florets
- 2 carrots, sliced thinly
- 1 small red onion, chopped
- 1 x 6 oz. pack of frozen pea pods, thaw before use
- 1 x 8 oz. can of sliced water chestnuts, not drained
- 4 cups of plain water
- 2 tbsps. of cornstarch
- 2 tsps. of white sugar
- 6 tbsps. of soy sauce
- 1/4 cup of white wine
- 1 tbsp. of fresh ginger, minced
- 1 tbsp. of vegetable oil
- 1 cup of Chinese cabbage, shredded
- 2 x large Bok choy heads, roughly chopped
- 1 tbsp. of vegetable oil

Instructions

1. Cook the brown rice according to directions, which should be around 50 minutes when the liquid has been absorbed.

2. In a small mixing bowl, add the cornstarch, soy sauce, sugar, and wine. Stir until all mixed, and you have a creamy paste

3. Stir in the minced ginger. Add the beef and cover all sides.

4. In a large skillet on medium-high heat, add 1 tbsp of oil.

5. Add the broccoli, carrots, onion, and the pea pods. Stir and cook for 1 minute.

6. Add the water chestnuts, cabbage, and bok choy. Cover the skillet and cook on a simmer for around 4 minutes until the vegetables are tender. Remove from the skillet but keep warm.

7. Using the same skillet over medium to high heat. Add and heat 1 tbsp of oil. Add the beef and cook until the desired likeness. 2 minutes each side for rare, or longer for well done.

8. Once the beef is cooked, add the warm vegetables into the skillet. Continue cooking for around 3 minutes until they are all heated.

9. Serve immediately over rice.

Meatless Shepherd's Pie

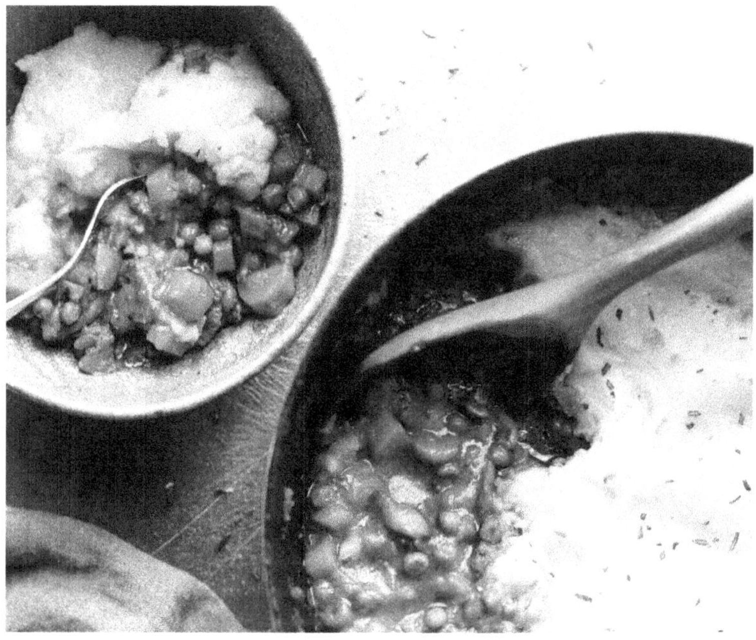

For a hearty dish that is as filling as much as it is tasty, this vegetarian classic shepherd's pie will please anyone. Just whip up a bowl full of gravy and this is a complete meal all on its own. The unique taste of marmite makes this dish something unlike any other fare of a similar nature.

Serving Size: 8

Preparation: 15 minutes

Cooking Time: 60 minutes

Ingredients

- 1/4 cup of dried pearl barley
- 1/2 cup of dry lentils
- 3 large potatoes, chopped
- 1 large carrot, roughly diced
- 2 cups of vegetable broth, divided into 2
- 1 tsp. of yeast extract, e.g. Marmite or alternative
- 1/2 medium onion, finely chopped
- 1/2 cup of chopped walnuts
- 1 tsp. of all-purpose flour
- 1/2 tsp. of water
- Sea salt and ground black pepper for taste

Instructions

1. Preheat the oven to 350 degrees Fahrenheit.

2. Place a large saucepan on low to medium heat. Add 1 1/4 cups of the broth, yeast extract, barley, and lentils — Cook for 30 minutes on a simmer.

3. In a separate medium saucepan, add the remaining 3/4 cup of broth. Add the carrots, onions, and walnuts. Cook for around 15 minutes or until tender.

4. Boil a large pot of salted water. Add the potatoes and cook for around 15 minutes until tender drain and mash.

5. Mix the flour and water in a small bowl then stir into the carrot mixture. Simmer the mixture until it thickens.

6. Mix both the carrot and lentil mixture — taste and season with sea salt and black pepper.

7. Add the mixture to a 2 x quart casserole dish. Scoop the mashed potatoes across the top of the lentil mixture.

8. Bake in the preheated oven for around 30 minutes until the top browns lightly.

9. Serve warm.

Desserts

Guilt-Free Banana Cake

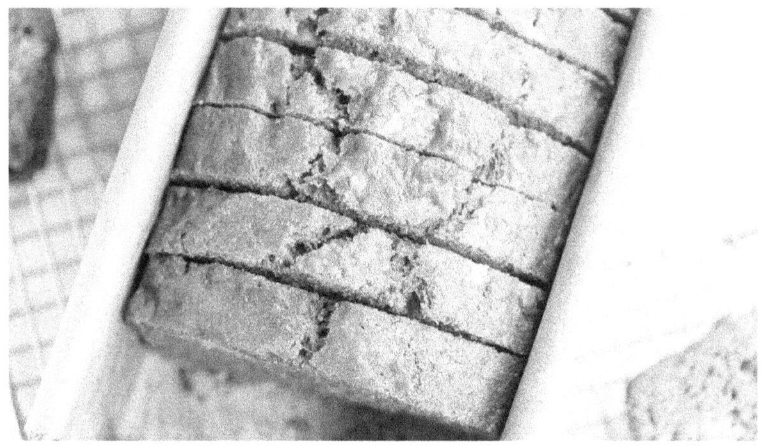

With ripe bananas delivering the sweetness, you can indulge in this quick and easy banana cake recipe and have a slice as a healthy dessert without feeling guilty. While it does use a package cake mix, this doesn't mean it is going to raise your cholesterol.

Serves: 24 Slices

Preparation: 15 minutes

Cooking Time: 60 minutes

Ingredients:

- 1 x 18.25 oz. pack of yellow ready-made cake mix
- 2 large bananas, very ripe and smashed
- 1 tsp. of baking soda

Instructions:

1. Follow the pack directions to make the mixture in a bowl. Do not cook yet.

2. In a separate bowl, add the baking soda to the peeled bananas and smash with a fork.

3. Add to the cake mix and stir to combine.

4. Oil and lightly flour a 9 x 13-inch baking tin and then pour the batter in. Tap gently to remove air bubbles.

5. Place the uncooked cake mix into a cold oven. Turn it on and set it to 350 degrees Fahrenheit

6. Bake for 60 minutes, a toothpick should come out clean at this point.

7. Let the cake before placing it in the refrigerator or topping with whipped cream.

Sugarless Oatmeal Cookie Bites

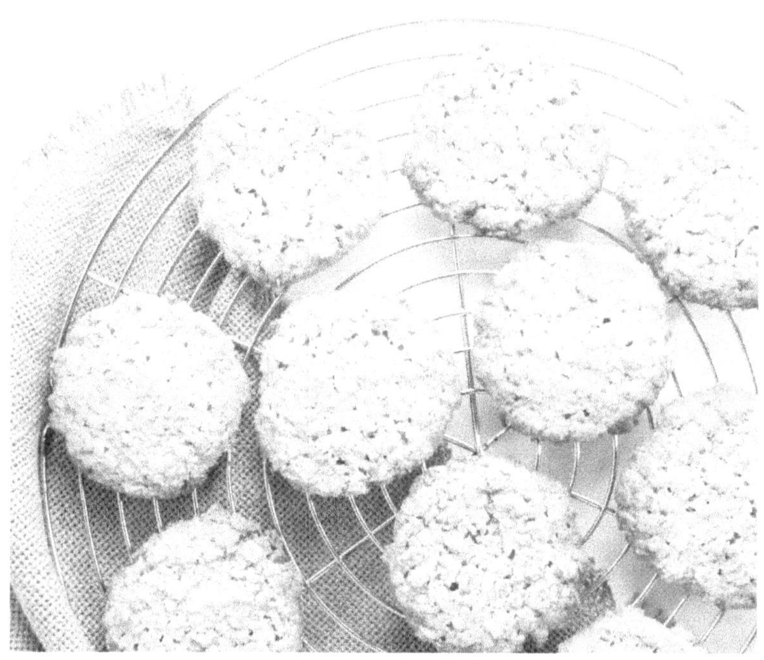

If you fancy something sweet after a healthy meal, then try one or two of these healthy oatmeal cookies that are sugar-free. When you want to keep your cholesterol down, these can make a great ending to any family dinner, or a late snack, and even a mid-morning treat.

Serves: 24

Preparation: 10 minutes

Cooking Time: 25 minutes

Ingredients:

- 2 cups of rolled oats
- 3 large bananas, very ripe and mashed
- 1/3 cup of applesauce, unsweetened
- 1/2 cup of raisins
- 1/4 cup of almond milk
- 1 tsp. of vanilla extract
- 1 tsp. of ground cinnamon

Instructions:

1. Preheat your oven to 350 degrees Fahrenheit.

2. In a large mixing bowl, add the oats, bananas, milk, raisins, vanilla extract, and cinnamon mix well until combined.

3. Lightly grease a nonstick baking sheet and cover with baking paper.

4. Place spoonful's of the mixture onto the sheet, leaving space for them to spread.

5. Bake for around 15 to 20 minutes in the middle of the oven until the edges brown lightly.

Sorbet a La Mango

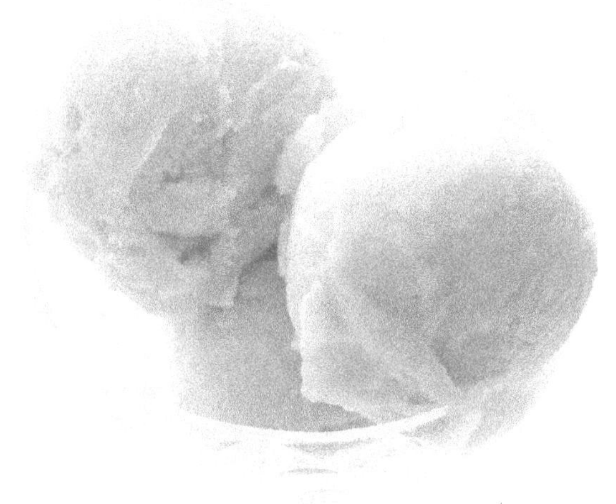

All it takes to make this super refreshing dessert is three **Ingredients**. With fresh mangos, a little syrup, and zesty lime juice, this is close enough to ice cream that will please any kid in the family. It only takes fifteen minutes to prepare and fifteen to chill, so even if you are in a rush, there is no reason not to indulge your sweet tooth.

Serves: 12

Preparation: 15 minutes

Cooking Time: 15 minutes

Ingredients:

- 4 large ripe mangoes – peel, remove seed and dice
- 1 cup of simple syrup
- 3 tbsps. of fresh lime-juice

Instructions:

1. Add the cubes of mango into a food processor or blender. Puree until smooth.

2. Add in the syrup and the juice of the lime. Puree until mixed and smooth

3. Add into an ice cream maker and freeze

Pumpkin Pudding Parfait

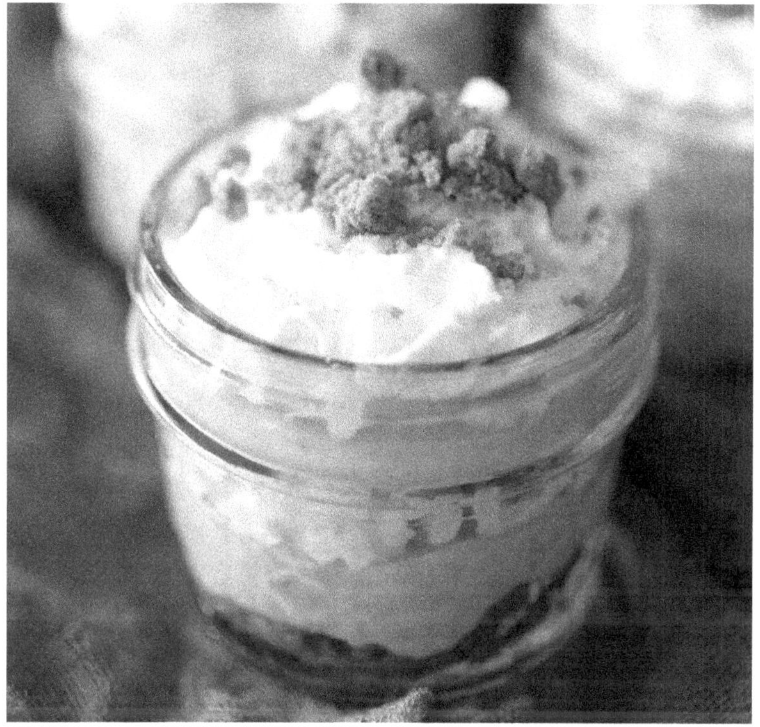

With the holiday season, there is no reason not to indulge. Here is a simple dessert that can hide the fact you are watching your cholesterol levels. It can be made in very little time and will have everyone guessing at what the **Ingredients** are. Even the kids will enjoy the taste.

Serves: 6

Preparation: 15 minutes

Cooking Time: 0 minutes

Ingredients:

- 1 cup of pureed pumpkin
- 1 x 1 oz. pack of sugar-free instant vanilla pudding
- 1 tsp. of pumpkin pie spices
- 1 cup of skimmed milk
- 1 cup of skimmed evaporated milk

Instructions:

1. In a large mixing bowl, add the puree, pudding mix, and the pie spice with the kinds of milk.

2. Use a blender and mix until thick and creamy

3. Spoon into dessert glasses or small bowls

4. Chill until set and ready to eat – top with whipped cream if desired

Conclusion

Many cookbooks need you to strip out all your **Ingredients** to purchase specific things. Our low cholesterol recipes use all you have in your pantry and refrigerator, so there is no need to think about increasing your grocery bill.

There may be one or two things to purchase, such as an exotic spice, yet these are long-lasting and will never be a waste.

Low cholesterol recipes are not as dull as you can see from the ones in this book. Every one of the low cholesterol recipes delivers plenty of fiber, omega 3-fatty acids, and lots of nutrients and vitamins. As a weight control program, every one of these cholesterol-reducing recipes will leave you satisfied.

You may find some are a hit with the kids of the house. Not one recipe is made with reducing cholesterol in mind as the objective, each of these delicious low cholesterol recipes was put together to taste fantastic first.

With all these, you need to take control of your eating habits, and the easiest way to do so is to work your way through this low cholesterol recipe book. Mix and match, and before you know it, you will have eaten yourself healthy.